Name of Look

Evening ○
Daytime ○

Face
Moisturizer

Concealer

Foundation

Highlight/Blush

Eyes
Brows

Eyelid

Liner

Crease

Mascara

Lips
Liner

Lip Color

Gloss

Notes

Name of Look _____

Evening ◯
Daytime ◯

Face
Moisturizer
_____

Concealer
_____

Foundation
_____

Highlight/Blush
_____

Eyes
Brows
_____

Eyelid
_____

Liner
_____

Crease
_____

Mascara
_____

Lips
Liner
_____

Lip Color
_____

Gloss
_____

Notes

Name of Look _____

Evening ○
Daytime ○

Face
Moisturizer
_____

Concealer
_____

Foundation
_____

Highlight/Blush
_____

Eyes
Brows
_____

Eyelid
_____

Liner
_____

Crease
_____

Mascara
_____

Lips
Liner
_____

Lip Color
_____

Gloss
_____

Notes

Name of Look _____

Evening ○
Daytime ○

Face
Moisturizer
_____

Concealer
_____

Foundation
_____

Highlight/Blush
_____

Eyes
Brows
_____

Eyelid
_____

Liner
_____

Crease
_____

Mascara

Lips
Liner
_____

Lip Color
_____

Gloss
_____

Notes

Name of Look _____

Evening ○
Daytime ○

Face
Brows
Moisturizer
_____

Concealer
_____

Foundation
_____

Highlight/Blush
_____

Eyes
Brows
_____

Eyelid
_____

Liner
_____

Crease
_____

Mascara
_____

Lips
Liner
_____

Lip Color
_____

Gloss
_____

Notes

Name of Look _____

Evening ○
Daytime ○

Face
Moisturizer
_____

Concealer
_____

Foundation
_____

Highlight/Blush
_____

Eyes
Brows
_____

Eyelid
_____

Liner
_____

Crease
_____

Mascara
_____

Lips
Liner
_____

Lip Color
_____

Gloss
_____

Notes

Name of Look _____

Evening ○
Daytime ○

Face
Moisturizer
_____

Concealer
_____

Foundation
_____

Highlight/Blush
_____

Eyes
Brows
_____

Eyelid
_____

Liner
_____

Crease
_____

Mascara

Lips
Liner
_____

Lip Color
_____

Gloss
_____

Notes

Name of Look _____

Evening ◯
Daytime ◯

Face
Moisturizer
_____

Concealer
_____

Foundation
_____

Highlight/Blush
_____

Eyes
Brows
_____

Eyelid
_____

Liner
_____

Crease
_____

Mascara

Lips
Liner
_____

Lip Color
_____

Gloss
_____

Notes

Name of Look _____

Evening ○
Daytime ○

Face
Moisturizer
_____

Concealer
_____

Foundation
_____

Highlight/Blush
_____

Eyes
Brows
_____

Eyelid
_____

Liner
_____

Crease
_____

Mascara
_____

Lips
Liner
_____

Lip Color
_____

Gloss
_____

Notes

Name of Look _____

Evening ⊙
Daytime ○

Face
Moisturizer
_____

Concealer
_____

Foundation
_____

Highlight/Blush
_____

Eyes
Brows
_____

Eyelid
_____

Liner
_____

Crease
_____

Mascara
_____

Lips
Liner
_____

Lip Color
_____

Gloss
_____

Notes

Name of Look _____

Evening ○
Daytime ○

Face
Moisturizer
_____

Concealer
_____

Foundation
_____

Highlight/Blush
_____

Eyes
Brows
_____

Eyelid
_____

Liner
_____

Crease
_____

Mascara
_____

Lips
Liner
_____

Lip Color
_____

Gloss
_____

Notes

Name of Look _____

Evening ○
Daytime ○

Face
Moisturizer
_____

Concealer
_____

Foundation
_____

Highlight/Blush
_____

Eyes
Brows
_____

Eyelid
_____

Liner
_____

Crease
_____

Mascara
_____

Lips
Liner
_____

Lip Color
_____

Gloss
_____

Notes

Name of Look _____

Evening ○
Daytime ○

Face
Moisturizer
_____

Concealer
_____

Foundation
_____

Highlight/Blush
_____

Eyes
Brows
_____

Eyelid
_____

Liner
_____

Crease
_____

Mascara
_____

Lips
Liner
_____

Lip Color
_____

Gloss
_____

Notes

Name of Look _____

Evening ○
Daytime ○

Face
Moisturizer

Concealer

Foundation

Highlight/Blush

Eyes
Brows

Eyelid

Liner

Crease

Mascara

Lips
Liner

Lip Color

Gloss

Notes

Name of Look _____

Evening ○
Daytime ○

Face
Moisturizer
_____

Concealer
_____

Foundation
_____

Highlight/Blush
_____

Eyes
Brows
_____

Eyelid
_____

Liner
_____

Crease
_____

Mascara
_____

Lips
Liner
_____

Lip Color
_____

Gloss
_____

Notes

Name of Look _____

Evening ⃝
Daytime ⃝

Face
Moisturizer

Concealer

Foundation

Highlight/Blush

Eyes
Brows

Eyelid

Liner

Crease

Mascara

Lips
Liner

Lip Color

Gloss

Notes

Name of Look _____

Evening ○
Daytime ○

Face
Moisturizer
_____

Concealer
_____

Foundation
_____

Highlight/Blush
_____

Eyes
Brows
_____

Eyelid
_____

Liner
_____

Crease
_____

Mascara
_____

Lips
Liner
_____

Lip Color
_____

Gloss
_____

Notes

Name of Look _____

Evening ○
Daytime ○

Face
Moisturizer
_____

Concealer
_____

Foundation
_____

Highlight/Blush
_____

Eyes
Brows
_____

Eyelid
_____

Liner
_____

Crease
_____

Mascara

Lips
Liner
_____

Lip Color
_____

Gloss
_____

Notes

Name of Look _____

Evening ○
Daytime ○

Face

Moisturizer
_____

Concealer
_____

Foundation
_____

Highlight/Blush
_____

Eyes

Brows
_____

Eyelid
_____

Liner
_____

Crease
_____

Mascara
_____

Lips

Liner
_____

Lip Color
_____

Gloss
_____

Notes

Name of Look _____

Evening ○
Daytime ○

Face
Moisturizer
_____

Concealer
_____

Foundation
_____

Highlight/Blush
_____

Eyes
Brows
_____

Eyelid
_____

Liner
_____

Crease
_____

Mascara
_____

Lips
Liner
_____

Lip Color
_____

Gloss
_____

Notes

Name of Look _____

Evening ◯
Daytime ◯

Face
Moisturizer
_____

Concealer
_____

Foundation
_____

Highlight/Blush
_____

Eyes
Brows
_____

Eyelid
_____

Liner
_____

Crease
_____

Mascara

Lips
Liner
_____

Lip Color
_____

Gloss
_____

Notes

Name of Look _____

Evening ○
Daytime ○

Face
Moisturizer
_____

Concealer
_____

Foundation
_____

Highlight/Blush
_____

Eyes
Brows
_____

Eyelid
_____

Liner
_____

Crease
_____

Mascara

Lips
Liner
_____

Lip Color
_____

Gloss
_____

Notes

Name of Look _____

Evening ○
Daytime ○

Face
Moisturizer
_____

Concealer
_____

Foundation
_____

Highlight/Blush
_____
_____

Eyes
Brows
_____

Eyelid
_____

Liner
_____

Crease
_____

Mascara
_____
_____

Lips
Liner
_____

Lip Color
_____

Gloss
_____

Notes

Name of Look _____

Evening ○
Daytime ○

Face
Moisturizer

Concealer

Foundation

Highlight/Blush

Eyes
Brows

Eyelid

Liner

Crease

Mascara

Lips
Liner

Lip Color

Gloss

Notes

Name of Look _____

Evening ○
Daytime ○

Face
Moisturizer
_____

Concealer
_____

Foundation
_____

Highlight/Blush
_____

Eyes
Brows
_____

Eyelid
_____

Liner
_____

Crease
_____

Mascara
_____

Lips
Liner
_____

Lip Color
_____

Gloss
_____

Notes

Name of Look _____

Evening ◯
Daytime ◯

Face
Moisturizer

Concealer

Foundation

Highlight/Blush

Eyes
Brows

Eyelid

Liner

Crease

Mascara

Lips
Liner

Lip Color

Gloss

Notes

Name of Look _____

Evening ○
Daytime ○

Face
Moisturizer
_____

Concealer
_____

Foundation
_____

Highlight/Blush
_____

Eyes
Brows
_____

Eyelid
_____

Liner
_____

Crease
_____

Mascara

Lips
Liner
_____

Lip Color
_____

Gloss
_____

Notes

Name of Look _____

Evening ○
Daytime ○

Face
Moisturizer
_____

Concealer
_____

Foundation
_____

Highlight/Blush
_____

Eyes
Brows
_____

Eyelid
_____

Liner
_____

Crease
_____

Mascara
_____

Lips
Liner
_____

Lip Color
_____

Gloss
_____

Notes

Name of Look _____

Evening ○
Daytime ○

Face
Moisturizer
_____

Concealer
_____

Foundation
_____

Highlight/Blush
_____

Eyes
Brows
_____

Eyelid
_____

Liner
_____

Crease
_____

Mascara
_____

Lips
Liner
_____

Lip Color
_____

Gloss
_____

Notes

Name of Look _____

Evening ○
Daytime ○

Face
Moisturizer
_____

Concealer
_____

Foundation
_____

Highlight/Blush
_____

Eyes
Brows
_____

Eyelid
_____

Liner
_____

Crease
_____

Mascara

Lips
Liner
_____

Lip Color
_____

Gloss
_____

Notes

Name of Look _____

Evening ○
Daytime ○

Face
Moisturizer
_____

Concealer
_____

Foundation
_____

Highlight/Blush
_____

Eyes
Brows
_____

Eyelid
_____

Liner
_____

Crease
_____

Mascara
_____

Lips
Liner
_____

Lip Color
_____

Gloss
_____

Notes

Name of Look _____

Evening ○
Daytime ○

Face
Moisturizer
_____

Concealer
_____

Foundation
_____

Highlight/Blush
_____
_____

Eyes
Brows
_____

Eyelid
_____

Liner
_____

Crease
_____

Mascara
_____

Lips
Liner
_____

Lip Color
_____

Gloss
_____

Notes

Name of Look _____

Evening ○
Daytime ○

Face
Moisturizer
_____

Concealer
_____

Foundation
_____

Highlight/Blush
_____

Eyes
Brows
_____

Eyelid
_____

Liner
_____

Crease
_____

Mascara
_____

Lips
Liner
_____

Lip Color
_____

Gloss
_____

Notes

Name of Look _____

Evening ○
Daytime ○

Face
Moisturizer
_____

Concealer
_____

Foundation
_____

Highlight/Blush
_____

Eyes
Brows
_____

Eyelid
_____

Liner
_____

Crease
_____

Mascara

Lips
Liner
_____

Lip Color
_____

Gloss

Notes

Name of Look _____

Evening ○
Daytime ○

Face
Moisturizer
_____

Concealer
_____

Foundation
_____

Highlight/Blush
_____

Eyes
Brows
_____

Eyelid
_____

Liner
_____

Crease
_____

Mascara
_____

Lips
Liner
_____

Lip Color
_____

Gloss
_____

Notes

Name of Look _____

Evening ○
Daytime ○

Face
Moisturizer
_____

Concealer
_____

Foundation
_____

Highlight/Blush
_____

Eyes
Brows
_____

Eyelid
_____

Liner
_____

Crease
_____

Mascara
_____

Lips
Liner
_____

Lip Color
_____

Gloss
_____

Notes

Name of Look _____

Evening ○
Daytime ○

Face
Moisturizer
_____

Concealer
_____

Foundation
_____

Highlight/Blush
_____

Eyes
Brows
_____

Eyelid
_____

Liner
_____

Crease
_____

Mascara
_____

Lips
Liner
_____

Lip Color
_____

Gloss
_____

Notes

Name of Look _____

Evening ◉
Daytime ○

Face
Moisturizer

Concealer

Foundation

Highlight/Blush

Eyes
Brows

Eyelid

Liner

Crease

Mascara

Lips
Liner

Lip Color

Gloss

Notes

Name of Look _____

Evening ○
Daytime ○

Face
Moisturizer
_____

Concealer
_____

Foundation
_____

Highlight/Blush
_____

Eyes
Brows
_____

Eyelid
_____

Liner
_____

Crease
_____

Mascara
_____

Lips
Liner
_____

Lip Color
_____

Gloss
_____

Notes

Name of Look _____

Evening ○
Daytime ○

Face
Moisturizer

Concealer

Foundation

Highlight/Blush

Eyes
Brows

Eyelid

Liner

Crease

Mascara

Lips
Liner

Lip Color

Gloss

Notes

Name of Look _____

Evening ○
Daytime ○

Face
Moisturizer
_____

Concealer
_____

Foundation
_____

Highlight/Blush
_____

Eyes
Brows
_____

Eyelid
_____

Liner
_____

Crease
_____

Mascara
_____

Lips
Liner
_____

Lip Color
_____

Gloss
_____

Notes

Name of Look _____

Evening ⊙
Daytime ○

Face
Moisturizer

Concealer

Foundation

Highlight/Blush

Eyes
Brows

Eyelid

Liner

Crease

Mascara

Lips
Liner

Lip Color

Gloss

Notes

Name of Look _____

Evening ◯
Daytime ◯

Face
Moisturizer
_____

Concealer
_____

Foundation
_____

Highlight/Blush
_____

Eyes
Brows
_____

Eyelid
_____

Liner
_____

Crease
_____

Mascara
_____

Lips
Liner
_____

Lip Color
_____

Gloss
_____

Notes

Name of Look _____

Evening ○
Daytime ○

Face
Moisturizer

Concealer

Foundation

Highlight/Blush

Eyes
Brows

Eyelid

Liner

Crease

Mascara

Lips
Liner

Lip Color

Gloss

Notes

Name of Look _____

Evening ○
Daytime ○

Face
Moisturizer
_____

Concealer
_____

Foundation
_____

Highlight/Blush
_____

Eyes
Brows
_____

Eyelid
_____

Liner
_____

Crease
_____

Mascara
_____

Lips
Liner
_____

Lip Color
_____

Gloss
_____

Notes

Name of Look _____

Evening ○
Daytime ○

Face
Moisturizer
_____

Concealer
_____

Foundation
_____

Highlight/Blush
_____

Eyes
Brows
_____

Eyelid
_____

Liner
_____

Crease
_____

Mascara
_____

Lips
Liner
_____

Lip Color
_____

Gloss
_____

Notes

Name of Look _____

Evening ○
Daytime ○

Face
Moisturizer
_____

Concealer
_____

Foundation
_____

Highlight/Blush
_____
_____

Eyes
Brows
_____

Eyelid
_____

Liner
_____

Crease
_____

Mascara
_____

Lips
Liner
_____

Lip Color
_____

Gloss
_____

Notes

Name of Look _____

Evening ○
Daytime ○

Face
Moisturizer
_____

Concealer
_____

Foundation
_____

Highlight/Blush
_____

Eyes
Brows
_____

Eyelid
_____

Liner
_____

Crease
_____

Mascara
_____

Lips
Liner
_____

Lip Color
_____

Gloss
_____

Notes

Name of Look _____

Evening ○
Daytime ○

Face
Moisturizer
_____

Concealer
_____

Foundation
_____

Highlight/Blush
_____

Eyes
Brows
_____

Eyelid
_____

Liner
_____

Crease
_____

Mascara
_____

Lips
Liner
_____

Lip Color
_____

Gloss
_____

Notes

Name of Look _____

Evening ○
Daytime ○

Face
Moisturizer
_____

Concealer
_____

Foundation
_____

Highlight/Blush
_____

Eyes
Brows
_____

Eyelid
_____

Liner
_____

Crease
_____

Mascara
_____

Lips
Liner
_____

Lip Color
_____

Gloss
_____

Notes

Name of Look _____

Evening ○
Daytime ○

Face
Moisturizer
_____

Concealer
_____

Foundation
_____

Highlight/Blush
_____

Eyes
Brows
_____

Eyelid
_____

Liner
_____

Crease
_____

Mascara
_____

Lips
Liner
_____

Lip Color
_____

Gloss
_____

Notes

Name of Look _____

Evening ◯
Daytime ◯

Face
Moisturizer
_____

Concealer
_____

Foundation
_____

Highlight/Blush
_____

Eyes
Brows
_____

Eyelid
_____

Liner
_____

Crease
_____

Mascara

Lips
Liner
_____

Lip Color
_____

Gloss
_____

Notes

Name of Look _____

Evening ○
Daytime ○

Face
Moisturizer
_____

Concealer
_____

Foundation
_____

Highlight/Blush
_____

Eyes
Brows
_____

Eyelid
_____

Liner
_____

Crease
_____

Mascara
_____

Lips
Liner
_____

Lip Color
_____

Gloss
_____

Notes

Name of Look _____

Evening ○
Daytime ○

Face
Moisturizer
_____

Concealer
_____

Foundation
_____

Highlight/Blush
_____

Eyes
Brows
_____

Eyelid
_____

Liner
_____

Crease
_____

Mascara
_____

Lips
Liner
_____

Lip Color
_____

Gloss
_____

Notes

Name of Look _____

Evening ○
Daytime ○

Face
Moisturizer
_____

Concealer
_____

Foundation
_____

Highlight/Blush
_____

Eyes
Brows
_____

Eyelid
_____

Liner
_____

Crease
_____

Mascara

Lips
Liner
_____

Lip Color
_____

Gloss
_____

Notes

Name of Look _____

Evening ○
Daytime ○

Face
Moisturizer
_____

Concealer
_____

Foundation
_____

Highlight/Blush
_____

Eyes
Brows
_____

Eyelid
_____

Liner
_____

Crease
_____

Mascara
_____

Lips
Liner
_____

Lip Color
_____

Gloss
_____

Notes

Name of Look _____

Evening ○
Daytime ○

Face
Moisturizer
_____

Concealer
_____

Foundation
_____

Highlight/Blush
_____

Eyes
Brows
_____

Eyelid
_____

Liner
_____

Crease
_____

Mascara
_____

Lips
Liner
_____

Lip Color
_____

Gloss
_____

Notes

Name of Look _____

Evening ⊙
Daytime ○

Face
Moisturizer

Concealer

Foundation

Highlight/Blush

Eyes
Brows

Eyelid

Liner

Crease

Mascara

Lips
Liner

Lip Color

Gloss

Notes

Name of Look _____

Evening ○
Daytime ○

Face
Moisturizer
_____

Concealer
_____

Foundation
_____

Highlight/Blush
_____

Eyes
Brows
_____

Eyelid
_____

Liner
_____

Crease
_____

Mascara
_____

Lips
Liner
_____

Lip Color
_____

Gloss
_____

Notes

Name of Look _____

Evening ○
Daytime ○

Face
Moisturizer
_____

Concealer
_____

Foundation
_____

Highlight/Blush
_____
_____

Eyes
Brows
_____

Eyelid
_____

Liner
_____

Crease
_____

Mascara
_____

Lips
Liner
_____

Lip Color
_____

Gloss
_____

Notes

Name of Look _____

Evening ○
Daytime ○

Face

Moisturizer
_____

Concealer
_____

Foundation
_____

Highlight/Blush
_____

Eyes

Brows
_____

Eyelid
_____

Liner
_____

Crease
_____

Mascara
_____

Lips

Liner
_____

Lip Color
_____

Gloss
_____

Notes

Name of Look _____

Evening ○
Daytime ○

Face
Moisturizer
_____

Concealer
_____

Foundation
_____

Highlight/Blush
_____

Eyes
Brows
_____

Eyelid
_____

Liner
_____

Crease
_____

Mascara

Lips
Liner
_____

Lip Color
_____

Gloss
_____

Notes

Name of Look _____

Evening ○
Daytime ○

Face
Moisturizer
_____

Concealer
_____

Foundation
_____

Highlight/Blush
_____

Eyes
Brows
_____

Eyelid
_____

Liner
_____

Crease
_____

Mascara
_____

Lips
Liner
_____

Lip Color
_____

Gloss
_____

Notes

Name of Look _____

Evening ○
Daytime ○

Face
Moisturizer
_____

Concealer
_____

Foundation
_____

Highlight/Blush
_____

Eyes
Brows
_____

Eyelid
_____

Liner
_____

Crease
_____

Mascara
_____

Lips
Liner
_____

Lip Color
_____

Gloss
_____

Notes

Name of Look _____

Evening ○
Daytime ○

Face
Moisturizer
_____

Concealer
_____

Foundation
_____

Highlight/Blush
_____

Eyes
Brows
_____

Eyelid
_____

Liner
_____

Crease
_____

Mascara

Lips
Liner
_____

Lip Color
_____

Gloss
_____

Notes

Name of Look _____

Evening ○
Daytime ○

Face
Moisturizer
_____

Concealer
_____

Foundation
_____

Highlight/Blush
_____

Eyes
Brows
_____

Eyelid
_____

Liner
_____

Crease
_____

Mascara

Lips
Liner
_____

Lip Color
_____

Gloss
_____

Notes

Name of Look _____

Evening ○
Daytime ○

Face
Moisturizer
_____

Concealer
_____

Foundation
_____

Highlight/Blush
_____

Eyes
Brows
_____

Eyelid
_____

Liner
_____

Crease
_____

Mascara
_____

Lips
Liner
_____

Lip Color
_____

Gloss
_____

Notes

Name of Look _____

Evening ○
Daytime ○

Face
Moisturizer
_____

Concealer
_____

Foundation
_____

Highlight/Blush
_____

Eyes
Brows
_____

Eyelid
_____

Liner
_____

Crease
_____

Mascara

Lips
Liner
_____

Lip Color
_____

Gloss

Notes

Name of Look _____

Evening ○
Daytime ○

Face

Moisturizer
_____

Concealer
_____

Foundation
_____

Highlight/Blush
_____

Eyes

Brows
_____

Eyelid
_____

Liner
_____

Crease
_____

Mascara
_____

Lips

Liner
_____

Lip Color
_____

Gloss
_____

Notes

Name of Look _____

Evening ○
Daytime ○

Face
Moisturizer
_____

Concealer
_____

Foundation
_____

Highlight/Blush
_____

Eyes
Brows
_____

Eyelid
_____

Liner
_____

Crease
_____

Mascara
_____

Lips
Liner
_____

Lip Color
_____

Gloss
_____

Notes

Name of Look _____

Evening ○
Daytime ○

Face
Moisturizer
_____

Concealer
_____

Foundation
_____

Highlight/Blush
_____

Eyes
Brows
_____

Eyelid
_____

Liner
_____

Crease
_____

Mascara

Lips
Liner
_____

Lip Color
_____

Gloss
_____

Notes

Name of Look _____

Evening ○
Daytime ○

Face
Moisturizer
_____

Concealer
_____

Foundation
_____

Highlight/Blush
_____

Eyes
Brows
_____

Eyelid
_____

Liner
_____

Crease
_____

Mascara

Lips
Liner
_____

Lip Color
_____

Gloss
_____

Notes

Name of Look _____

Evening ○
Daytime ○

Face

Moisturizer

Concealer

Foundation

Highlight/Blush

Eyes

Brows

Eyelid

Liner

Crease

Mascara

Lips

Liner

Lip Color

Gloss

Notes

Name of Look _____

Evening ○
Daytime ○

Face
Moisturizer
_____

Concealer
_____

Foundation
_____

Highlight/Blush
_____

Eyes
Brows
_____

Eyelid
_____

Liner
_____

Crease
_____

Mascara

Lips
Liner
_____

Lip Color
_____

Gloss
_____

Notes

Name of Look _____

Evening ○
Daytime ○

Face
Moisturizer
_____

Concealer
_____

Foundation
_____

Highlight/Blush
_____

Eyes
Brows
_____

Eyelid
_____

Liner
_____

Crease
_____

Mascara
_____

Lips
Liner
_____

Lip Color
_____

Gloss
_____

Notes

Name of Look _____

Evening ○
Daytime ○

Face
Moisturizer

Concealer

Foundation

Highlight/Blush

Eyes
Brows

Eyelid

Liner

Crease

Mascara

Lips
Liner

Lip Color

Gloss

Notes

Name of Look _____

Evening ○
Daytime ○

Face

Moisturizer
_____

Concealer
_____

Foundation
_____

Highlight/Blush
_____

Eyes

Brows
_____

Eyelid
_____

Liner
_____

Crease
_____

Mascara
_____

Lips

Liner
_____

Lip Color
_____

Gloss
_____

Notes

Name of Look _____

Evening ○
Daytime ○

Face
Moisturizer
_____

Concealer
_____

Foundation
_____

Highlight/Blush
_____
_____

Eyes
Brows
_____

Eyelid
_____

Liner
_____

Crease
_____

Mascara
_____

Lips
Liner
_____

Lip Color
_____

Gloss
_____

Notes

Name of Look _____

Evening ○
Daytime ○

Face
Moisturizer
_____

Concealer
_____

Foundation
_____

Highlight/Blush
_____

Eyes
Brows
_____

Eyelid
_____

Liner
_____

Crease
_____

Mascara

Lips
Liner
_____

Lip Color
_____

Gloss

Notes

Name of Look _____

Evening ○
Daytime ○

Face
Moisturizer
_____

Concealer
_____

Foundation
_____

Highlight/Blush
_____

Eyes
Brows
_____

Eyelid
_____

Liner
_____

Crease
_____

Mascara
_____

Lips
Liner
_____

Lip Color
_____

Gloss
_____

Notes

Name of Look _____

Evening ○
Daytime ○

Face
Moisturizer
_____

Concealer
_____

Foundation
_____

Highlight/Blush
_____

Eyes
Brows
_____

Eyelid
_____

Liner
_____

Crease
_____

Mascara
_____

Lips
Liner
_____

Lip Color
_____

Gloss
_____

Notes

Name of Look _____

Evening ○
Daytime ○

Face
Moisturizer

Concealer

Foundation

Highlight/Blush

Eyes
Brows

Eyelid

Liner

Crease

Mascara

Lips
Liner

Lip Color

Gloss

Notes

Name of Look _____

Evening ○
Daytime ○

Face
Moisturizer

Concealer

Foundation

Highlight/Blush

Eyes
Brows

Eyelid

Liner

Crease

Mascara

Lips
Liner

Lip Color

Gloss

Notes

Name of Look _____

Evening ○
Daytime ○

Face
Moisturizer
_____

Concealer
_____

Foundation
_____

Highlight/Blush
_____

Eyes
Brows
_____

Eyelid
_____

Liner
_____

Crease
_____

Mascara
_____

Lips
Liner
_____

Lip Color
_____

Gloss
_____

Notes

Name of Look _____

Evening ○
Daytime ○

Face
Moisturizer
_____

Concealer
_____

Foundation
_____

Highlight/Blush
_____

Eyes
Brows
_____

Eyelid
_____

Liner
_____

Crease
_____

Mascara
_____

Lips
Liner
_____

Lip Color
_____

Gloss
_____

Notes

Name of Look _____

Evening ○
Daytime ○

Face
Moisturizer
_____

Concealer
_____

Foundation
_____

Highlight/Blush
_____

Eyes
Brows
_____

Eyelid
_____

Liner
_____

Crease
_____

Mascara

Lips
Liner
_____

Lip Color
_____

Gloss
_____

Notes

Name of Look _____

Evening ○
Daytime ○

Face
Moisturizer
_____

Concealer
_____

Foundation
_____

Highlight/Blush
_____

Eyes
Brows
_____

Eyelid
_____

Liner
_____

Crease
_____

Mascara
_____

Lips
Liner
_____

Lip Color
_____

Gloss
_____

Notes

Name of Look _____

Evening ⊙
Daytime ○

Face
Moisturizer
_____

Concealer
_____

Foundation
_____

Highlight/Blush
_____

Eyes
Brows
_____

Eyelid
_____

Liner
_____

Crease
_____

Mascara

Lips
Liner
_____

Lip Color
_____

Gloss
_____

Notes

Name of Look _____

Evening ○
Daytime ○

Face
Moisturizer
_____

Concealer
_____

Foundation
_____

Highlight/Blush
_____

Eyes
Brows
_____

Eyelid
_____

Liner
_____

Crease
_____

Mascara
_____

Lips
Liner
_____

Lip Color
_____

Gloss
_____

Notes

Name of Look _____

Evening ○
Daytime ○

Face
Moisturizer
_____

Concealer
_____

Foundation
_____

Highlight/Blush
_____

Eyes
Brows
_____

Eyelid
_____

Liner
_____

Crease
_____

Mascara

Lips
Liner
_____

Lip Color
_____

Gloss
_____

Notes

Name of Look _____

Evening ○
Daytime ○

Face
Moisturizer
_____

Concealer
_____

Foundation
_____

Highlight/Blush
_____

Eyes
Brows
_____

Eyelid
_____

Liner
_____

Crease
_____

Mascara
_____

Lips
Liner
_____

Lip Color
_____

Gloss
_____

Notes

Name of Look _____

Evening ○
Daytime ○

Face
Moisturizer
_____

Concealer
_____

Foundation
_____

Highlight/Blush
_____

Eyes
Brows
_____

Eyelid
_____

Liner
_____

Crease
_____

Mascara
_____

Lips
Liner
_____

Lip Color
_____

Gloss
_____

Notes

Name of Look _____

Evening ○
Daytime ○

Face
Moisturizer
_____

Concealer
_____

Foundation
_____

Highlight/Blush
_____

Eyes
Brows
_____

Eyelid
_____

Liner
_____

Crease
_____

Mascara
_____

Lips
Liner
_____

Lip Color
_____

Gloss
_____

Notes

Name of Look _____

Evening ○
Daytime ○

Face
Moisturizer
_____

Concealer
_____

Foundation
_____

Highlight/Blush
_____

Eyes
Brows
_____

Eyelid
_____

Liner
_____

Crease
_____

Mascara

Lips
Liner
_____

Lip Color
_____

Gloss
_____

Notes

Name of Look _____

Evening ○
Daytime ○

Face
Moisturizer
_____

Concealer
_____

Foundation
_____

Highlight/Blush
_____

Eyes
Brows
_____

Eyelid
_____

Liner
_____

Crease
_____

Mascara
_____

Lips
Liner
_____

Lip Color
_____

Gloss
_____

Notes

Name of Look _____

Evening ○
Daytime ○

Face
Moisturizer
_____

Concealer
_____

Foundation
_____

Highlight/Blush
_____

Eyes
Brows
_____

Eyelid
_____

Liner
_____

Crease
_____

Mascara
_____

Lips
Liner
_____

Lip Color
_____

Gloss
_____

Notes

Name of Look _____

Evening ◯
Daytime ◯

Face

Moisturizer
_____

Concealer
_____

Foundation
_____

Highlight/Blush
_____

Eyes

Brows
_____

Eyelid
_____

Liner
_____

Crease
_____

Mascara
_____

Lips

Liner
_____

Lip Color
_____

Gloss
_____

Notes

Name of Look _____

Evening ○
Daytime ○

Face
Moisturizer
_____

Concealer
_____

Foundation
_____

Highlight/Blush
_____

Eyes
Brows
_____

Eyelid
_____

Liner
_____

Crease
_____

Mascara

Lips
Liner
_____

Lip Color
_____

Gloss

Notes

Name of Look _____

Evening ○
Daytime ○

Face
Moisturizer
_____

Concealer
_____

Foundation
_____

Highlight/Blush
_____

Eyes
Brows
_____

Eyelid
_____

Liner
_____

Crease
_____

Mascara
_____

Lips
Liner
_____

Lip Color
_____

Gloss
_____

Notes

Name of Look _____

Evening ○
Daytime ○

Face
Moisturizer
_____

Concealer
_____

Foundation
_____

Highlight/Blush
_____

Eyes
Brows
_____

Eyelid
_____

Liner
_____

Crease
_____

Mascara

Lips
Liner
_____

Lip Color
_____

Gloss
_____

Notes

Name of Look _____

Evening ○
Daytime ○

Face
Moisturizer
_____

Concealer
_____

Foundation
_____

Highlight/Blush
_____

Eyes
Brows
_____

Eyelid
_____

Liner
_____

Crease
_____

Mascara
_____

Lips
Liner
_____

Lip Color
_____

Gloss
_____

Notes

Name of Look _____

Evening ○
Daytime ○

Face
Moisturizer
_____

Concealer
_____

Foundation
_____

Highlight/Blush
_____

Eyes
Brows
_____

Eyelid
_____

Liner
_____

Crease
_____

Mascara
_____

Lips
Liner
_____

Lip Color
_____

Gloss
_____

Notes

Name of Look _____

Evening ◯
Daytime ◯

Face

Moisturizer
_____

Concealer
_____

Foundation
_____

Highlight/Blush
_____

Eyes

Brows
_____

Eyelid
_____

Liner
_____

Crease
_____

Mascara
_____

Lips

Liner
_____

Lip Color
_____

Gloss
_____

Notes

Name of Look _____

Evening ○
Daytime ○

Face
Moisturizer
_____

Concealer
_____

Foundation
_____

Highlight/Blush
_____

Eyes
Brows
_____

Eyelid
_____

Liner
_____

Crease
_____

Mascara

Lips
Liner
_____

Lip Color
_____

Gloss
_____

Notes

Name of Look _____

Evening ◯
Daytime ◯

Face
Moisturizer
_____

Concealer
_____

Foundation
_____

Highlight/Blush
_____

Eyes
Brows
_____

Eyelid
_____

Liner
_____

Crease
_____

Mascara
_____

Lips
Liner
_____

Lip Color
_____

Gloss
_____

Notes

Name of Look _____

Evening ◉
Daytime ○

Face
Moisturizer

Concealer

Foundation

Highlight/Blush

Eyes
Brows

Eyelid

Liner

Crease

Mascara

Lips
Liner

Lip Color

Gloss

Notes

Name of Look _____

Evening ○
Daytime ○

Face
Moisturizer
_____

Concealer
_____

Foundation
_____

Highlight/Blush
_____

Eyes
Brows
_____

Eyelid
_____

Liner
_____

Crease
_____

Mascara
_____

Lips
Liner
_____

Lip Color
_____

Gloss
_____

Notes

Name of Look _____

Evening ◯
Daytime ◯

Face
Moisturizer

Concealer

Foundation

Highlight/Blush

Eyes
Brows

Eyelid

Liner

Crease

Mascara

Lips
Liner

Lip Color

Gloss

Notes

Name of Look _____

Evening ○
Daytime ○

Face
Moisturizer
_____

Concealer
_____

Foundation
_____

Highlight/Blush
_____

Eyes
Brows
_____

Eyelid
_____

Liner
_____

Crease
_____

Mascara
_____

Lips
Liner
_____

Lip Color
_____

Gloss
_____

Notes

Name of Look _____

Evening ◯
Daytime ◯

Face
Moisturizer
_____

Concealer
_____

Foundation
_____

Highlight/Blush
_____

Eyes
Brows
_____

Eyelid
_____

Liner
_____

Crease
_____

Mascara
_____

Lips
Liner
_____

Lip Color
_____

Gloss
_____

Notes

Name of Look _____

Evening ○
Daytime ○

Face
Moisturizer
_____

Concealer
_____

Foundation
_____

Highlight/Blush
_____

Eyes
Brows
_____

Eyelid
_____

Liner
_____

Crease
_____

Mascara
_____

Lips
Liner
_____

Lip Color
_____

Gloss
_____

Notes

Name of Look _____

Evening ○
Daytime ○

Face
Moisturizer
_____

Concealer
_____

Foundation
_____

Highlight/Blush
_____

Eyes
Brows
_____

Eyelid
_____

Liner
_____

Crease
_____

Mascara
_____

Lips
Liner
_____

Lip Color
_____

Gloss
_____

Notes

Name of Look _____

Evening ○
Daytime ○

Face
Moisturizer

Concealer

Foundation

Highlight/Blush

Eyes
Brows

Eyelid

Liner

Crease

Mascara

Lips
Liner

Lip Color

Gloss

Notes

Name of Look _____

Evening ○
Daytime ○

Face
Moisturizer
_____

Concealer
_____

Foundation
_____

Highlight/Blush
_____

Eyes
Brows
_____

Eyelid
_____

Liner
_____

Crease
_____

Mascara
_____

Lips
Liner
_____

Lip Color
_____

Gloss
_____

Notes

Name of Look _____

Evening ○
Daytime ○

Face
Moisturizer
_____

Concealer
_____

Foundation
_____

Highlight/Blush
_____

Eyes
Brows
_____

Eyelid
_____

Liner
_____

Crease
_____

Mascara
_____

Lips
Liner
_____

Lip Color
_____

Gloss
_____

Notes

Name of Look _____

Evening ○
Daytime ○

Face
Moisturizer
_____

Concealer
_____

Foundation
_____

Highlight/Blush
_____

Eyes
Brows
_____

Eyelid
_____

Liner
_____

Crease
_____

Mascara

Lips
Liner
_____

Lip Color
_____

Gloss
_____

Notes

Name of Look _____

Evening ○
Daytime ○

Face
Moisturizer
_____

Concealer
_____

Foundation
_____

Highlight/Blush
_____

Eyes
Brows
_____

Eyelid
_____

Liner
_____

Crease
_____

Mascara
_____

Lips
Liner
_____

Lip Color
_____

Gloss
_____

Notes

Name of Look _____

Evening ○
Daytime ○

Face
Moisturizer
_____

Concealer
_____

Foundation
_____

Highlight/Blush
_____

Eyes
Brows
_____

Eyelid
_____

Liner
_____

Crease
_____

Mascara
_____

Lips
Liner
_____

Lip Color
_____

Gloss
_____

Notes

Name of Look _____

Evening ○
Daytime ○

Face
Liner
_____

Concealer
_____

Foundation
_____

Highlight/Blush
_____

Eyes
Brows
_____

Eyelid
_____

Liner
_____

Crease
_____

Mascara
_____

Lips
Liner
_____

Lip Color
_____

Gloss
_____

Notes

Name of Look _____

Evening ○
Daytime ○

Face
Moisturizer
_____

Concealer
_____

Foundation
_____

Highlight/Blush
_____

Eyes
Brows
_____

Eyelid
_____

Liner
_____

Crease
_____

Mascara
_____

Lips
Liner
_____

Lip Color
_____

Gloss
_____

Notes

www.ingramcontent.com/pod-product-compliance
Lightning Source LLC
LaVergne TN
LVHW012119070526
838202LV00056B/5779